NATURAL CURE FOR TYPE 2 DIABETES

A One-Of-A-Kind Book to Help Treat and Reverse Type 2 Diabetes.

RS Johnson

DEDICATION

Dedicated to my wife and my 4 lovely children

CONTENTS

CHAPTER 8: THE BEST NATURAL "DRUGS" FOR TYPE 2 DIABETES AT THE CELLULAR LEVEL 39

CHAPTER 9: THE BEST NATURAL INSULIN FOR TYPE 2 DIABETES 44

CHAPTER 10: WHAT ARE THE BEST HEALTH SUPPLEMENTS FOR TYPE 2 DIABETES?

CHAPTER 11: DIET FOR TYPE 2 DIABETES

CHAPTER 12: EXERCISE AND DIABETES

ACKNOWLEDGMENTS

To My Family

INTRODUCTION

What is Diabetes?

Type 1 diabetes is an autoimmune illness, signifying that your immune system attacks and destroys the cells in your pancreas that make insulin. This usually happens over a few days or weeks.

Type 2 diabetes develops when the insulin-producing cells don't work as well as they should or when the cells don't produce enough insulin. It most often starts slowly and gets worse over time, although if you have prediabetes, it can happen quickly.

The cells of your muscles and your fat tissue don't respond well to insulin. This is known as insulin resistance. Insulin resistance usually starts before you notice symptoms of Diabetes and can lead to type 2 diabetes.

With both types, the amount of sugar or glucose in your blood rises above normal levels.

Individuals with prediabetes are at great danger of developing type 2 diabetes, especially if they have a family history of the disease.

Do I have prediabetes?

The only way to know for sure if you have prediabetes is to get tested. A test requiring an overnight fast followed by blood tests is the most accurate.

There's an increased risk for cardiovascular disease if you have prediabetes, and low-risk interventions can help prevent complications.

But to know your true risk, you need to make lifestyle changes.

Action Steps: Lower Blood Sugar Levels

Even if you aren't sure whether your blood sugar levels are too high, it's always best to lower them by eating properly and being active. Here are some ways to do that:

- Eat at minimum half of your everyday grains as whole grains.
- Eat at least four servings of fresh fruit and vegetables each day.
- Choose lean meats such as poultry, which is lower in saturated fat than

red meat (beef, pork).

- Choose low-fat dairy products such as skim milk and fat-free or low-fat yogurt.
- Limit foods high in grains.

If you need to lose weight, be sure you don't starve yourself or eat so little that your blood sugar levels go too low (hypoglycemia). You should eat no less than a 1,200-calorie diet.

Exercise and Watch Your Style of Eating

Even if you've been told that you have type 2 diabetes, you can still take steps to control blood sugar. Here are some tips:

- Don't skip meals anywhere near bedtime.
- Avoid sugary foods and drinks since they can raise blood sugar levels unexpectedly.
- Take frequent low-dose insulin before meals or snacks if your blood sugar levels are high, not because it controls your blood sugar level but because taking it with food keeps the insulin from raising your blood sugar too much.
- Watch your weight, and work with a dietitian to create a diet that is right for you.
- Exercise for at least 30 minutes most days of the week.

Prediabetes is the "grey area" or transition period leading to type 2 diabetes. People with prediabetes may not have any symptoms, but if left untreated, people with prediabetes are likely to develop type 2 diabetes within ten years. They will often require oral medication (pills). If those do not work due to side effects or ineffectiveness, insulin shots will be required if low blood sugar is dealt with effectively and consistently.

In 2006, an estimated 54 million people in the U.S. had prediabetes. This number represents 15.5% of the U.S. population. Of those individuals with prediabetes, 29 million had full-blown type 2 diabetes (53%), and 26 million had prediabetes (47%).

Research in endocrinology has also attempted to find the biological mechanism behind a high-fat diet causing weight gain. However, although it was found that saturated fat raises levels of LDL cholesterol, it is still not entirely clear why it would raise one's risk for health problems like obesity and heart disease.

This book will help you understand what type 2 diabetes is and how to naturally cure it.

CHAPTER 1:
WHAT IS TYPE 2 DIABETES?

Type 2 Diabetes is a long-lasting illness that disturbs the way you body uses sugar. People with Type 2 Diabetes need to maintain a healthy balanced diet and take action when their blood glucose level rises.

Type 1 and Type 2 Diabetes: Similarities and Differences

Type 1 and Type 2 Diabetes differ from each other in many ways First, there is no cure for Type 2 diabetes. Also, people with Type 2 diabetes have a little more control over their insulin levels because insulin can be made in the body. However, it is mostly controlled by the pancreas that does not work properly or does not work in severe type 2 diabetes. On the other hand, five hormones are needed to function properly, and these hormones cannot be produced by the body of someone with type 2 diabetes (despite taking insulin).

Type 2 Diabetes: More Than Just High Blood Glucose

In addition to high blood sugar, people with Type 2 diabetes may also develop some of the following symptoms:

Fatigue and Weakness

Fatigue is a prevalent symptom of Type 2 diabetes. It can be caused by not sleeping enough or medications that suppress the central nervous system. Fear, anxiety, depression, and stress also contribute to fatigue. Fatigue can result in major problems for someone with Type 2 diabetes as it may make it hard for them to do daily tasks such as cooking and cleaning. They may also experience pain caused by nerve damage from glucose deposits throughout the body.

Wants to EAT

People suffering from Type 2 diabetes often feel hungry. As a result they may consume more than the recommended number of calories each day. Furthermore, they may eat high sugar content such as cookies, cakes, candy, soda pop and ice cream. They also tend to eat nutrient-poor foods such as chocolate and pastries, containing many saturated fat and refined carbohydrates. These high-sugar foods are not good for someone with Type 2 diabetes as these foods do not provide any real nutritional value and contain no fibre. Also, these foods can cause a spike in blood glucose levels.

Is Tired of Taking Medications

Some people with Type 2 diabetes do not like taking medications to control their blood glucose levels. Some of these drugs include biguanides (Metformin), alpha-glucosidase inhibitors (Acarbose), and thiazolidinediones (Rosiglitazone and Pioglitazone). These drugs can be the reason for numerous side effects that make it difficult for the person to stay motivated to take them. Some of these side effects include upset stomach, gas, diarrhea, or weight gain. Fatigue is another common side effect of some of these drug classes, including biguanides and thiazolidinediones. To make matters worse, these drugs are also known to cause other health problems such as low HDL cholesterol, elevated liver enzymes, and kidney damage.

Doesn't Feel Well

People with type 2 diabetes may also experience repeated infections. They may also have a feeling of uneasiness. They may feel that their hair looks greyer, or they are gaining weight out of the ordinary. Some people with Type 2 diabetes even feel a constant feeling of hunger without eating anything at all.

Type 2 Diabetes in the USA

In the United States, over 26 million people are now living with diabetes mellitus. Of this number, 55 per cent have Type 2 diabetes. It is also estimated that 86 million Americans are pre-diabetics, and another 29 million of those pre-diabetics do not even know they are pre-diabetics. With these numbers on the rise, obesity in the US is also on the rise. In 2004, it was estimated that two-thirds of American adults were either overweight or obese. The total number of obese people in the US has risen to over 20 per cent, equating to 36 million people.

The normal age of beginning for Type 2 diabetes is 47 years old. It is most prevalent between the ages of 45-64. 40 per cent of people who have 5.6 times the pre-diabetic risk in 20 years or less will develop

Diabetes within that time. And, half of those people with 8.5 times higher risk will develop Diabetes within 14 years or less than half as long as those with 5.6 times higher risk!

It was forecast that the figure of cases of Diabetes mellitus would rise by 50 per cent by 2010 and 75 per cent by 2020. However, the prevalence of Diabetes worldwide already exceeds that projected. Some other experts have said that by 2040, the number of cases of type 1 diabetes will double annually, and the number of cases of type 2 diabetes will triple!

The main cause for prediabetes is overweight. When a person's body becomes accustomed to having a constant supply of glucose (sugar) for energy, either through eating carbohydrate-rich foods or by storing excess glucose as fat, his/her pancreas no longer produces enough insulin to properly function.

CHAPTER 2:
WHAT THE SYMPTOMS OF DIABETES LOOKS LIKE

Diabetes is a chronic health condition that affects approximately 8% of the US population and 25% of people aged 65 years and older. Every year, between 140,000–230,000 people die because of diabetes-related complications. The warning signs for Diabetes usually come as follows:

Excessive Thirst or Frequent Urination

An individual who is thirsty incessantly and has to urinate often should be concerned about whether or not they have Diabetes. They are most likely suffering from something other than Diabetes.

Excessive Hunger

Patients can suffer from excessive hunger and need to eat frequently. For this reason, even if they are quite thin, they do not look healthy like someone who is healthy and has normal blood sugar levels.

Fatigue

An individual suffering from Diabetes will feel very tired after a meal or after exercise. "Tired" does not mean that the individual needs to rest; it means that their blood sugar level is too low, and it will make them tired after a while even if they did nothing at all else than eating or exercising normally.

Fatigue, as a symptom of Diabetes, can be confused with extreme tiredness due to other conditions. For example, it may be due to a common cold or gastroenteritis.

Working professionals who are going through stressful periods can suffer from fatigue and sudden exhaustion in the early morning hours. It can also occur if the individual does not get enough sleep. The cause of this symptom cannot necessarily be determined with just a blood-sugar test; therefore, it does not mean that this person has Diabetes.

Frequent Night Falls

People who experience night falls and restlessness easily in the evening hours may be suffering from either Diabetes or hypoglycemia. Sometimes, sleep disturbances are also associated with depression and other psychological problems. If the person falls asleep right after meals and does not fall asleep afterwards, then they might very well be suffering from hypoglycemia.

Diabetes-Related Perspiration

Some people experience sweating even when they do not exercise and feel very high body temperature. This may be a symptom of hypoglycemia or hyperglycemia, but it might result from another condition. If you believe that you experience excessive sweating without any other explanation, then you should consult a medical professional to determine how to address your symptoms.

Anxiety

A person suffering from Diabetes may feel anxious and not want to go out of their home. They might also experience shaking or even sweating before a stressful event. This is very common, and it is usually caused because of the high or low levels of blood sugar in the body. It is not necessarily an indication of Diabetes, but it may indicate that they struggle with hypoglycemia.

Joint Pain

A person suffering from Diabetes might experience pain when exercising. It does not mean they should stop exercising; it could also be because they have arthritis, but it is most likely due to the multitude of symptoms that come with poorly controlled blood sugar levels.

Sudden Weight Gain

People who are overweight can easily lose weight if they are just getting started, but as they lose more, the calories being burned begin to slow down. This causes fat to be stored in other areas, and thus the person may experience sudden weight gain. If you have been working out and eating accurately regularly before experiencing this sudden gain, then you might be suffering from undiagnosed Diabetes.

In Growing Toenails

Suppose a person is unable to get rid of their ingrown toenails due to Diabetes or hypoglycemia. In that case, it is a sign that something else is seriously wrong with their glucose levels. It could be time to speak with your doctor and find out if you are suffering from Diabetes.

Skin Infections

People who are diabetic have a hard time fighting off infections. They do not heal as fast from wounds, and they also experience skin that is easily susceptible to infections. You may want to have a higher intake of vitamin C, which can be found in citrus fruits like oranges, lemons, and grapefruits. If it gets too bad, you might want to consider antibiotics because they can help clear up any lingering infections that can cause further disruption in your life and progress.

Diabetes is a serious disorder that distresses your body's ability to produce or use insulin correctly. It can be dangerous for people who are diabetic.

While the warning signs above are almost universal, the symptoms they bring about are somewhat personal and may vary from each individual. For every characteristic of high blood sugar, there is a physical outcome that may follow.

Although high blood sugar is common, most people with Diabetes do not have ketoacidosis. Many diabetics do well if their blood glucose levels are kept at normal levels. Since untreated Diabetes can destroy the body over time, it is important to take steps to prevent or reduce the risk of long-term complications such as kidney disease and nerve damage. This requires close monitoring of blood sugars (triglycerides and cholesterol as well) and closely supervising any diabetic medication actions such as insulin dosage level, etc., for the benefit of overall health.

Symptoms and signs of hyperglycemia can be alleviated by the correction of the condition that causes it. This signifies that if you have Diabetes and hypoglycemia, then make sure to seek the help of a medical professional.

Although hypoglycemia is an extremely common condition in diabetics, it is very important to get it treated as soon as possible because of the serious long-term consequences of its untreated state.

How Is Diabetes Diagnosed?

Diabetes can be diagnosed via blood test, a sleep study

(polysomnogram), or in some states with a urine test (fasting glucose).
This method can be used especially if your symptoms fit into one of the
categories listed above: excessive thirst, anxiety, fatigue, frequent night
falls or weight gain.

Numerous tests can be completed to diagnose Diabetes. They include:

- Blood test: Your blood will be tested for sugar level (glucose and other types of sugar).

- Glucose tolerance test (GTT): A blood sample is drawn, and glucose is given intravenously. You will have to fast, and then the next day another blood sample will be drawn. Your blood sugar increases after you eat. The higher the number, the better your response. The normal glucose level for an 80-year-old is 100 or below. The range should be between 70 - 130 mg/dl before breakfast and 95 - 140 mg/dl after meals.

- Random blood sugar test: A blood sample is taken without regard to meals or exercise. Around 140 mg/dl is normal, but the range should be between 70 - 130 mg/dl before breakfast and 95 - 140 mg/dl after meals.

- Oral glucose tolerance test (OGTT): This is a more comprehensive test used to diagnose Diabetes in children and pregnant women. It includes a fasting blood glucose level (not eating for up to 8 hours) then two blood sugar readings are taken after the patient has drunk a sugary solution.

Fasting plasma glucose (FPG): This test measures how much glucose is in your blood when you have not eaten in over 8 hours. A level of 100 or below is normal.

CHAPTER 3:
THE CAUSES OF DIABETES

The causes of Diabetes are complicated. There is not one single cause because a combination of factors can cause the condition. Diabetes is usually developed in adults over the age as a result of any number of factors. These are some of the causes of Diabetes

Infection

According to a research study on the connection between infection and the development of Diabetes, around 75% of all cases of Diabetes are caused by infections. Infections during the early stage can lead to the onset of Diabetes in patients.

Genetics

You only have one chance if you carry the gene for the condition. Diseases like sickle cell anaemia, Tay-Sachs and beta-thalassemia increase the risk of developing type 2 diabetes. You can inherit the disease from your mother or father. The risk is greater in families who have a history of Diabetes in their family.

The risk of developing Diabetes is higher among siblings and people with certain genetic backgrounds predisposing them to develop the disease. There is a greater chance for a person at risk to develop Diabetes if two or more people already have it among their family members.

When a parent or sibling is diabetic, you have a greater risk of developing type 2 diabetes than those whose relatives do not have the disease. It is important to know that there are many different types of Diabetes, so what makes type 1 different from type 2 may be how each person's body responds to glucose in their blood.

Obesity

Obesity can lead to type 2 diabetes. According to an international study, around seventy per cent of the people who are obese are at risk for developing Type 2 diabetes. It is a leading cause of Diabetes. In the United States alone, about one-third of the population suffers from obesity, and about twenty per cent have Diabetes.

Based on the National Centre for Health Statistics, almost half of American adults are overweight. That is because they have a body mass index greater than the normal level of 25-29.9. Studies have shown that people with obesity are about five times more likely to develop type 2 diabetes than those not obese. As little as 10-15 extra pounds on your frame can set off the development of this condition.

Age

Over fifty-five per cent of diabetic patients are at least sixty-five years old. Another thirty-five per cent are over forty and still developing the condition. Diabetes can also result from chronic conditions such as hypertension, gout, diverticulitis, early-stage kidney disease or polycystic ovary syndrome (PCOS). All these conditions can be risk factors for developing Diabetes. Genetics and family history can also be a factor in developing this condition

Birth Control Pills

The pills like desogestrel, norethindrone, and progestin have been linked to the development of Diabetes. The pills interfere with the woman's production of insulin.

Amount of Weight Gained During Pregnancy

A woman who gains thirty or more pounds during pregnancy is at risk for developing type 2 diabetes during the time after her pregnancy ends. The risk is greatest during the first six months after childbirth but can extend for up to five years from birth to their child.

Certain Physical Disorders

Certain conditions that affect the body and blood vessels, like peripheral vascular disease, can promote the development of Diabetes. Some of these illnesses include aplastic anaemia, chronic liver disease, sickle cell disease and viral encephalitis.

High-Risk Physical Activity

The greater the level of physical activity you engage in, the less likely you are to develop type 2 diabetes. However, if you engage in physical activity, it is important to make sure it is at a moderate pace and not too strenuous. You need to keep your intensity level around that of an average person's.

Certain Types of Cancer

Those with cancer, especially non-Hodgkins lymphoma, are more likely to develop type 2 diabetes than people without it. Research has shown that people with leukemia tend to develop Diabetes at a younger age than other people. The diseases affecting blood vessels also increase your chances of developing the condition.

Certain Medications

The use of certain medications can cause type 2 diabetes to develop in some people. These include glucocorticoids like prednisone and some antidepressants.

Pregnancy Diabetes

More than 50 per cent of mothers with gestational Diabetes go on to develop type 2 diabetes later in life. Gestational Diabetes develops when your body does not produce enough insulin or cannot process it effectively. If you have type 2 diabetes and become pregnant, your glucose levels will be monitored closely throughout. You may also need to take insulin after giving birth.

Smoking

Smoking increases the risk of Diabetes by 30 per cent. It also increases the risk of atherosclerosis, heart disease and stroke. The effect on blood glucose levels is not as clear, but research shows that smokers have an increase in all glycaemic markers. In addition, people who are obese or overweight on average have a 12-point higher glucose tolerance factor (GTF). This means that more insulin needs to be secreted by the pancreas to lower their blood glucose levels compared to those who are a healthy weight.

CHAPTER 4:
STAGES OF DIABETES

This talks about the stages of Diabetes and provides valuable information on preventing it from spiralling out of control. Different symptoms accompany different stages, but they all share a common denominator: steadily declining blood sugar levels, leading to more serious complications.

All of us need to understand that Diabetes is a chronic disease. The body develops it slowly, but over the years, a person with Diabetes will require more and more medical attention to manage the disease.

There are several treatment options for Diabetes that are available, but none of these is perfect. Different combinations of medications and lifestyle changes can effectively control blood sugar levels and prevent further complications associated with Diabetes. Diabetes should not be considered a death sentence or something that cannot be cured. Long-term control and the right attitude can keep a person alive as long as they don't ignore information on preventing complications from developing in their health condition such as blindness, kidney failure, heart attack, stroke and more.

Here are the stages of Diabetes:

Stage 1: Molecular (Insulin Resistance)

During this stage, it's already possible for the body to be resistant to insulin. The pancreas can still produce insulin; nevertheless, the body will start to require more of it as time goes by. When this happens, the pancreas starts to become overworked and eventually becomes less effective.

An individual in this stage should pay attention to the amount of physical activity that they are doing. If you have a hard time doing exercises that move your muscles and not your joints, you may want to switch these forms of exercises to make sure that your muscles get the necessary stimulation.

This is where taking pills can help control blood sugar levels in the body. A higher rate of weight gain also characterizes this stage. As for weight, an individual in this stage needs to keep a close watch on their body fat and their diet. This is the stage where a person with Diabetes should maintain healthy body fat and also make sure that the carbs they eat are properly broken down into glucose.

Stage 2: Biochemical Cardiometabolic Risk (Prediabetes)

The pancreas has been damaged in this stage, but it's still producing enough insulin to keep blood sugar levels in a normal range. An individual in this stage can develop type 2 diabetes if they don't take action. This is when dietary changes are vital. A diet of fruits, veggies and whole grains should be supplemented by exercise.

Several medications can control blood sugar levels during this stage, including Metformin and Actos and Glucophage and Glyburide. These are the only treatments that can prevent a person from developing type 2 diabetes.

At this stage, it's already possible for a person to develop type 2 diabetes because the body has already become fully resistant to insulin. The body is already producing less insulin than necessary, which makes up for its lack by consuming more glucose from other sources such as food and medications.

This is the stage where people should pay close attention to their diet. This is when eating healthy foods can be beneficial because you will get more oxygen to your cells and make your cells work better. Your liver will also produce more insulin if you eat healthy foods such as protein, vegetables, fruits and grains.

Stage 3: Biochemical Disease (Type 2 Diabetes)

Type 2 diabetes can impact any part of the body, but it is usually associated with chronic complications such as heart problems, kidney failure, nerve damage and stroke. Because blood sugar levels in this stage are not well-monitored, it can result in more serious complications. However, the best thing you can do is keep your blood sugar levels under control, so you don't have to suffer from other complications.

People with Diabetes usually experience weight loss, and this is because the body's cells are not receiving enough sugar from the blood. Even though this happens, the person's appetite does not decrease. This makes you want to eat more which means your calorie intake cannot be well-regulated even if your calorie output decreases. This imbalance makes you have Diabetes even if you have been eating healthy food.

Stage 4: Vascular Complications (Type 2 Diabetes with Complications)

This is the stage wherein Diabetes can result in serious problems such as blindness and amputations. However, these complications can be prevented as long as a person's blood sugar levels are under control. In this stage, the world is getting to know more and more about Diabetes even if you are unaware of it.

People in this stage should be educated about the dangers and health needs of good control of blood sugar levels. Diagnosis is very important in this stage because a person can be unaware of his/her condition and not take action to prevent it.

People can recover from type 2 diabetes only if they are diligent in suppressing their blood sugar levels. Once they are diagnosed with Diabetes, they need to monitor their blood glucose level frequently and give themselves insulin shots three times a week so that their body will not have too much glucose in the bloodstream.

If you have been told that you are at stage 3 or 4 of Diabetes, do not despair. You can still correct your condition through proper diet and exercise by following the advice from your physician. More than ever you need to watch your blood sugar level so you can take the necessary steps to help yourself get better.

Once you discover that you have Diabetes, it will be hard for you to think straight and think about the consequences of having Diabetes. It's normal for people with Diabetes to ignore or underestimate their condition because it doesn't seem bad.

However, as soon as Diabetes is not well-managed, it can result in more serious complications such as heart disease, which can cause a person to lose his/her life. The best thing that a person with type 2 diabetes can do is maintain a healthy lifestyle, so they don't have to suffer from other complications such as blindness and amputations.

CHAPTER 5:
HOW TO PREVENT TYPE 2 DIABETES

Diabetes is a disease that affects not only your heart and nervous system but also your digestive system. Here, we will explore the causes of and treatments for Type 2 diabetes.

Type 2 diabetes (T2DM) is an ongoing condition in which the body cannot regulate blood sugar levels properly. This means that glucose stays high in the bloodstream after a meal because insulin cannot lower it down to normal levels. The cells in your pancreas create less insulin or none at all to compensate for this problem, making T2DM more common with age.

T2DM can lead to nerve damage, blindness, kidney damage, heart disease, and even amputation in the most severe cases. These complications of Diabetes are sometimes referred to as 'diabetic complications'.

Consequently, what must you do to avert your body from developing Type 2 Diabetes?

Eat A Balanced Diet

Make sure you eat a well-balanced diet to help manage your Type 2 diabetes and prevent heart disease, stroke, and kidney disease complications. A healthy diet is rich in fruits and vegetables, whole grains, lean protein sources, and essential fats. Did you know that people who eat more fresh produce are also less likely to develop Type 2 diabetes?

Eating too much of any one thing can cause you to gain weight, leading to Diabetes. Eat a balanced diet that consists of fruits, vegetables, whole grains and lean proteins such as fish and chicken.

With Type 2 diabetes, we usually recommend bulking up on fibre-rich food like broccoli and cauliflower. Fibre not only helps you feel full but also helps regulate blood sugar levels, making it ideal for diabetics.

Also recommended in your diet are high-antioxidant foods like berries, apples, spinach and nuts. Antioxidants aid to fight free radicals that damage cells in your body. This will slow down the processes that lead to diabetes complications.

Lose Weight

As mentioned, carrying extra weight around your belly can also lead to insulin resistance. In a study published in the Journal of Clinical Endocrinology & Metabolism, researchers found that "the more fat you had inside your abdominal cavity, the less sensitive you were to insulin." So, losing belly fat will help you prevent Diabetes.

To do this, follow our simple weight loss tips:

- Eat a healthy breakfast every morning.
- Limit the amount of refined, processed and fast food you eat.
- Keep your daily caloric intake at an average of 2,000 calories per day or less.
- Stay active by walking, doing yoga or cycling for 30 minutes a day, five times a week.

We're forgoing our typical exercise advice this week because we think you should eat healthily first and then work out a second time for muscle toning. This will help avoid the 'skinny-fat look that some people get after doing hours of cardio without lifting weights.

Excess belly fat is associated with insulin resistance and Type 2 diabetes risk, so those of you who are overweight probably won't want to skip this week's tip! The key is to cut back on calories by eating small meals rather than large dinner meals throughout the day. Undertaking this will retain your blood sugar levels steady and help keep you from developing Type 2 diabetes.

Reducing Alcohol Intake

Alcohol has a great number of calories and can be the reason for a build-up of fat around your stomach. Also, beer and other boozy drinks are packed with sugar, which increases insulin levels in the body. So, if you're trying to reduce your risk of developing Type 2 diabetes, stay away from the booze!

Reduce Stress

Everyone experiences stressful situations at one point or another. It's important to remember that stress can trigger health problems, especially in those who already have Type 4 diabetes. So, try to learn how to handle daily stressors and reduce the amount of time you spend worrying about future problems.

Stop Smoking

For many people, cigarettes are an addiction. If you're reading this book and you still smoke, quit now! Smoking is a major risk factor for Type 2 diabetes. According to Diabetes.co.uk, smokers are twice as likely to develop the disease as non-smokers.

Lower Blood Pressure

Having high blood pressure can upsurge your danger of developing Type 2 diabetes. Consequently, make it a point to have your blood pressure checked regularly and take steps to control it.

Exercise

The 2007 Physical Activity Guidelines for Americans recommend regular physical activity for everyone. People with Diabetes, however, should check in with their doctors before starting any new exercise regimen. Start unhurriedly and slowly raise the length and intensity of your workouts to avoid any over-exertion.

Maintain a Healthy Weight

One of the greatest customs to avert Type 2 diabetes is to make sure you don't become overweight or obese. If you're already overweight, start eating healthier foods and engaging in more physical activity, so you can shed a few pounds. If you're healthy, make sure you don't gain extra pounds by eating healthy and exercising regularly.

Embrace all kinds of fruits and vegetables. Try not to place them in the refrigerator for too long as they will lose their nutrients. Try to eat 5 portions of fruit or veg a day: 3 fresh portions (ideally) plus 2 portions of dried fruit or canned veg. If you have trouble eating 5 portions, here are some ideas. Take in at minimum 1 portion of fruit or veg in each meal. The best types are whole fruits, not juices; raw vegetables; leafy green veg; and root veg. Vegetables contain fibre that helps lower cholesterol and blood glucose levels and be a source of non-animal protein that doesn't raise IGF-1 levels. Eat more beans, pulses, lentils or tofu to increase your protein intake and fill up with fewer calories.

In some cultures, beans may be considered a food group for their nutritional value but are mostly classified as "pulses" (along with lentils and peas. Although they contain unsaturated fat, pulses tend to be high in carbs and should not be eaten as a protein source (unless you're vegetarian or vegan). Beans can also be high in starch and sugars, which are not good for your heart, especially if you are a type 1 diabetic who has been diagnosed with prediabetes.

According to the American Diabetes Association (ADA), beans, peas or lentils high in fibre will help decrease the risk of Diabetes (type 2) by as much as 16-20%. So, include them in your diet.

Subsequently, this is meant for those who already have Type 2 diabetes or are at risk for developing it in the future, but if you don't fit into those categories and want to avoid getting Diabetes later in life anyway, follow these tips too! All of them will help keep your insulin levels under control and lower your blood sugar levels.

CHAPTER 6:
HOW TO REVERSE TYPE 2 DIABETES

What Does It Means to Reverse Type 2 Diabetes?

Type 2 diabetes is a metabolic disorder where the body cannot produce enough insulin to meet its needs. What does it mean to reverse type 2 diabetes? This would typically be a more difficult question than you might assume; however, many studies have demonstrated that diet and exercise can reverse this condition.

In one study, people who followed the diet showed improved levels of A1C, a common blood test for comparing how well you're controlling your blood sugar. Another study demonstrated reductions in waist circumference after changes in lifestyle habits were made as well as an improvement in insulin resistance scores during the same time frame. In other words, the alterations in diet and exercise resulted in positive changes for the participants in both studies.

In a study involving a very low-calorie diet, participants saw their weight significantly reduced, and their A1C levels lowered back to normal. As time goes on, more people report success at reversing their type 2 diabetes with diet and exercise. One interesting aspect of these studies is that the researcher's credit "the American Diabetes Association guidelines" for helping to keep the participants motivated enough to stick with it.

So, how to reverse type 2 diabetes?

Reduce Your Calorie Intake

According to the researchers, the American Diabetes Association guidelines for how much you should eat (to avoid developing type 2 diabetes) are outdated. They suggest that people consume about 1,400 calories per day, which is only if they're trying to gain weight. If you need to lose weight, then it's suggested that you consume about 1,200 calories per day. The most important thing is to keep track of your weight and try not to gain weight if it's causing you many problems.

If the American Diabetes Association guidelines aren't adequate for your needs, other options can help boost your chances of reversing type 2 diabetes.

Eat A Healthy Diet

Your diet plays a vast part in helping you lose weight, and in turn, it can help prevent your body from developing type 2 diabetes in the first place.

In a study where mice were given a high-fat diet, they developed type 2 diabetes within 15 weeks. However, when the mice had access to insulin over that same time, they didn't develop this disease. In other words, if you give your body too much sugar and fat, it will respond by developing Diabetes as a way to try to compensate for the extra calories that it's consuming.

Another study demonstrated just how powerful a simple lifestyle change could be in reversing type 2 diabetes. In this study, the patients were provided with a very low-calorie diet, and they experienced significant reductions in their blood glucose levels. After doing this for some time, they switched over to a low-fat diet, which resulted in ever greater improvements.

Try Supplementation

You may have overheard about the profits of taking certain supplements to help you lose weight, and in many cases, these supplements can play an important role in helping you reverse type 2 diabetes as well. One type of supplement that has been proposed for use in reversing type 2 diabetes is bromelain, also known as pineapple enzyme or papaya enzyme.

In a double-blind, placebo-controlled study, twenty pregnant women with gestational Diabetes were given either bromelain or a placebo, and their blood glucose was monitored over the next 16 weeks. The results showed that the patients who received bromelain had much lower blood glucose levels than those who received the placebo.

Take Regular Exercise

Exercise can play a significant part in assisting you to lose weight and in turn reversing type 2 diabetes. In a small study, one group of men was instructed to exercise regularly for six months before entering into a 6-

month exercise phase where they exercised twice per week at 80% of their max heart rate during those 6 months. The results showed that the men in the exercise group had better glucose tolerance than those not exercising.

Get Plenty of Sleep

Getting enough quality sleep is extremely important because it helps your body manage stress levels, repair and rejuvenate cells, and balance hormones, which are all important factors for reversing type 2 diabetes. Sleep deprivation doesn't just negatively affect those with Diabetes; it is bad for your overall health too. A recent study showed that participants who averaged less than 6 hours per night had a much greater risk of developing cardiovascular disease than those who got at least 8 hours per night.

The most important advice I can give concerning getting enough sleep is to prioritize it and eliminate stress as much as possible. This is particularly correct if you are sleeping less than 5 hours per night on average or have trouble falling asleep at night when trying to lose weight.

Don't get caught up in a vicious circle where skipping meals and exercising becomes part of your lifestyle.

Reduce Stress Levels Through Relaxation Techniques, Hobbies, Meditation or Prayer

Stress is a silent killer but can be very effectively managed through relaxation techniques. A study done by the University of California showed that meditation reduces blood sugar levels and improves insulin sensitivity.

Use Herbs and Spices Wisely to Increase Your Intake of Antioxidants

Antioxidants are some of your best allies in the fight against Diabetes, since they fight free radicals, which damage cells and tissues and increase inflammation in the body. Some important antioxidants include vitamin E, vitamin C, beta-carotene (a precursor to vitamin A) and selenium. Here and now is a good period to start using herbs and spices such as turmeric, coriander seeds, Cinnamon or black pepper.

Try Homeopathy to Help Manage Your Blood Sugar

Levels

Certain homeopathic remedies can help keep your blood sugar levels at an optimal level. These include Calcarea carbonica, Natrum muriaticum and Cuprum arsenicosum. Studies have demonstrated that there are many people with Diabetes who report good results from homeopathy in helping them manage their blood sugar levels and associated symptoms such as fatigue, weakness, anxiety, and depression.

Improve The Efficiency of Your Pancreas by Supplementing with Alpha Lipoic Acid (ALA)

ALA is an antioxidant that is important for healthy liver function. It further helps insulin become more efficient, which improves insulin's action on your cells. It also helps improve the effects of insulin in helping your cells use glucose.

ALA has been shown to improve the efficiency of insulin produced by the beta cells in your pancreas.

Try SAM-E or Melatonin Supplementation

A great number of studies prove that supplementing with therapeutic amounts of SAM-e and melatonin can help people who are suffering from Diabetes by improving their insulin sensitivity while increasing blood glucose levels and even reducing fat levels in the body.

Don't Skip Meals

It is very important that you don't skip meals, either because you think that you can or because it's a habit that you've fallen into. Skipping mealtimes can be the reason your blood sugar levels spike, which can be very dangerous for people with Diabetes.

CHAPTER 7:
THE NATURAL CURE FOR DIABETES

Many people suffer from Diabetes. It can be exasperating and tough to manage, but it doesn't have to be a life-long disease. There are natural cures for Diabetes that will help you regulate your blood sugar, increase your energy levels, and take control of your life. This is the ultimate guide to natural remedies for Diabetes.

Apple Cider Vinegar

Apple cider vinegar helps the body produce insulin and is therefore considered a great natural remedy for Diabetes.

Animal Protein

While protein, in general, can help increase your energy levels and regulate your blood sugar, animal protein is of greater benefit. Animal protein not only provides you with the complete balance of amino acids your body needs, but it also contains fewer carbohydrates, which are not easily burned by the diabetic body.

Garlic

Studies have revealed that individuals who eat garlic often have lower blood glucose levels than people who do not eat garlic. Garlic also has anticoagulant and anti-clotting properties that help prevent the formation of blood clots, which is another cause of Diabetes.

Ginger

Ginger is a top natural remedy for Diabetes. It has been scientifically established to aid lesser blood glucose levels and inhibit alpha-amylase, which degrades starch and sugar molecules into glucose. Ginger can be taken in extract or raw form. You can add fresh slices to food or drink ginger juice for a quick energy boost. Remember to exercise caution when using ginger because it has been known to lower blood pressure in some individuals, leading to dizziness or fainting when standing up too quickly.

Salmon

Salmon is an excellent source of protein and omega 3 fatty acids. Omega-3s are proven to reduce the rate of glucose absorption and thus help to regulate blood sugar. It can likewise be used as a natural remedy for Diabetes because it contains many nutrients that can help the body function at full capacity. This will increase energy levels, suppress appetite, improve heart health, and enhance immune function.

Tea

Camellia sinensis is a flowering plant in the family Malvaceae, native to China, that has been used for centuries as a remedy for Diabetes. The tea acts on the pancreas by reducing its activity and increasing its excretion (secretion). Research shows that drinking green tea can significantly lower blood glucose levels, increase insulin sensitivity and help to normalize blood sugar.

Wheatgrass

Wheatgrass is grass created by wheat and produced from the stalks and husks of wheat after steamed or baked. Wheatgrass contains vitamins, minerals, chlorophyll, antioxidants, and enzymes that can help stabilize blood sugar levels. It also contains chlorophyll which serves as an antioxidant so that glucose is not stored as fat but is used to fuel vital functions such as cell energy production.

Brazil Nuts

Brazil nuts are also known as abacates, sometimes called brazils. They are a fruit of the tropical rainforest tree of the same name and are grown in South America. Brazil nuts are rich in manganese, which is necessary for healthy glucose metabolism. Manganese is also an essential trace element that may be deficient in those with Diabetes.

Green Tea

Studies display that green tea might aid to regulate blood sugar levels. Furthermore, to be filled in antioxidants, green tea contains catechin, which can lower blood glucose levels by acting on the digestive tract and reducing alpha-amylase activity (break down of starch into sugar).

Kiwi Fruit

Kiwis are also known as Chinese gooseberries, and they are a fruit of the kiwi plant (Actinidia chinensis). They are filled with vitamin C and other antioxidants that help to increase blood glucose levels. The fruit is also a good source of potassium, which may help to reduce the risk of developing type 2 diabetes.

Oats

Oatmeal is a popular breakfast cereal made from rolled oats that have been steamed or cooked. Studies show that oats eaten with milk improve blood glucose levels, which may be due to their high content of B vitamins and fibre (which may help slow down digestion and control insulin release).

Pistachio Nuts

Pistachios are very popular nuts that come from the tree of the same name, which is related to cashew and mango trees. Pistachios are a great basis of vitamin B6, amino acid tryptophan, and fibre, which can help reduce blood glucose levels and prevent heart disease and Diabetes.

Olives

Olives are fruit from the olive tree (Olea europaea) with tasty black or green flesh around a wrinkly pit. They may help lower blood sugar by making cells more sensitive to insulin. They also contain polyphenols - an antioxidant that is thought to help alleviate inflammation associated with type 2 diabetes.

Olive Oil

Olive oil is popular cooking oil. It is one of the healthiest oils because it contains monounsaturated fats, reducing cholesterol and controlling blood sugar levels. It also contains vitamin E, which helps produce cholesterol-lowering hormones vital for healthy insulin levels.

Psyllium Husks

Psyllium Hous is an ancient remedy for Diabetes that dates back to ancient Egypt, where it was used to remedy diabetic ulcers. Psyllium reduces blood glucose levels by reducing the absorption rate of sugar by the digestive tract and the liver, which in turn produces more insulin and less glucose.

Salmon Liver Oil

Salmon liver oil is a type of fish oil rich in omega-3 fatty acids, such as eicosapentaenoic acid (EPA) and docosahexaenoic acid (DHA). These fats are shown to help decrease blood glucose levels by improving insulin sensitivity and decreasing insulin resistance. Additionally, salmon liver oil also contains vitamin A, which has anti-cancer properties that may reduce the risk of type 2 diabetes.

Spirulina

It is a blue-green alga that is one of the most nutritious foods available. Spirulina provides many nutrients to help your body absorb energy from food and prevent blood sugar levels from rising too high. I contains vitamin B12 and several amino acids, which are necessary for the production of energy-releasing hormones. It also contains a healthy balance of folic acid and can help prevent birth defects in pregnant women.

Soy Beans

Soybeans are an important source of protein, fibre, carbohydrates and minerals. Soybeans contain isoflavones that act on the liver by helping to produce insulin and lower blood sugar levels. They also contain phytoestrogens which may provide many health benefits by balancing female hormone levels, improving immune function and reducing the risk of developing type 2 diabetes in postmenopausal women.

Rice Bran

Rice bran is a nutritious outer layer that is removed from white rice during processing. It is rich in B vitamins and fibre, which can help your body to produce and maintain healthy hormone levels, reduce blood glucose levels, regulate bowel movements, improve digestion and protect against colon cancer.

Wheat Germ Oil

Wheat germ oil is extracted from the seeds of wheat plants with a hydraulic press or an expeller press. It is filled with vitamins A, D and E as well as essential fatty acids. It contains some potent antioxidant compounds that are important for the health of cells, tissues and organs including the liver and pancreas. Wheat germ oil can help your body produce insulin and lower blood glucose levels.

Whey Protein Powder

Whey protein comes from milk and contains all the essential amino acids your body needs to produce energy. It is particularly high in leucine, which increases muscle protein synthesis so that you have more energy for physical activities such as exercise or work.

CHAPTER 8:
THE BEST NATURAL "DRUGS" FOR TYPE 2 DIABETES AT THE CELLULAR LEVEL

Herbs can be a great substitute for prescription drugs when it comes to the treatment of Diabetes. Herbs have been used in the treatment of Diabetes for centuries, and new medical research has shown that some herbs can be just as effective at treating type 2 diabetes without any side effects.

Phytochemicals

Phytochemicals are found in plants and are responsible for fighting off illnesses such as Diabetes. These natural plant extracts can prevent the cells from becoming damaged by free radicals. They can also stop glycation (deterioration of cell proteins), restore youthful functioning of cell membranes, help to lower blood glucose levels and promote better liver function. One phytochemical can be taken orally or intravenously that has been studied in combination with metformin: Vitamin C. It has been revealed to advance insulin sensitivity without any side effects.

Here are the herbs that can help diabetes patients at the cellular level:

Turmeric

Turmeric is a powerful anti-inflammatory herb that is derived from the root of the Curcuma longa plant. In a study conducted by the Department of Biochemistry at the University of Michigan, it was discovered that curcumin (the active ingredient in turmeric) has a positive effect on glucose metabolism. It also demonstrated antioxidant, anti-glycating, and lipophilic effects. The Department of Natural Medicine at Tilak Maharashtra College of Ayurveda in India studied 65 patients with type 2 diabetes and compared them with healthy non-diabetic controls. The study showed that turmeric effectively controlled the blood sugar level in people with type 2 diabetes. One group of participants in the study were given 600 mg turmeric three times a day, while another group received 600 mg five times a day. It was found that blood sugar levels were brought down by an average of 9.25% in the folks who drank the ground root powder daily for six weeks.

Curcumin is a polyphenol that is accountable for much of the exceptional health benefits of turmeric. Curcumin stimulates cell regeneration and acts as an anti-inflammatory agent which helps reduce inflammation that leads to heart disease, cancer, arthritis, and diabetic complications.

Gymnema Sylvestre

Gymnema Sylvestre, a plant native to India, is another exceptional herb that has been used to treat type 2 diabetes in Ayurvedic medicine. The word "gymnema" means "destroyer of sugar" and is derived from the Greek word "γυμνήματος", which means sweet. GYM1 is a water-soluble extract derived from the leaf of the Gymnema plant that has been used in India for centuries as a herbal treatment for Diabetes. Interestingly, there are 100 diabetics per 1,000 population in India — yet they have one of the lowest rates of heart disease globally. GYM1 inhibits beta-amyloid peptide (Aβ) and prevents insulin-mediated glucose uptake in the tissues of diabetic animals. The Indian tradition of Ayurvedic medicine relies on herbs and regularly includes nutritional supplements for the treatment of Diabetes. A current study directed by the Indian Council of Medical Research in cooperation with Zebra Biomedical Research Laboratories, Inc. examined the effects of GYM1 on glucose levels in ADH gene expression. The study concluded that GYM1 could suppress ADH expression, which was associated with a reduction in blood glucose levels.

Alpha Lipoic Acid

Alpha-lipoic acid (ALA) is an essential fatty acid that acts as a potent antioxidant and functions as a coenzyme in glucose metabolism to produce energy. ALA was originally believed to be effective in treating Diabetes only when used with insulin, but recent studies have shown that it is equally beneficial for type 2 diabetics. A 2009 study published in the "Diabetes, Metabolic Syndrome and Obesity: Targets and Therapy" journal showed that ALA improves blood sugar control by its action on insulin resistance. Another German study conducted at the University of Leipzig concluded that ALA positively affects postprandial hyperglycemia in diabetic patients. Furthermore, an Italian study at the

University of Padua showed that ALA could reduce glycated haemoglobin levels in type 2 diabetics and healthy volunteers.

Cinnamon Extract

Cinnamon is a spice gotten from the inner bark of numerous trees belonging to the genus Cinnamomum. It has conventionally been utilized for its health benefits and antioxidant properties because it contains various bioactive compounds such as polyphenols, cinnamaldehyde, eugenol, and pulegone. Studies have shown that cinnamon extract exhibits blood sugar lowering potential because it stimulates insulin secretion and potentiates glucose uptake by cells. Moreover, Cinnamon reduces glycated haemoglobin levels and improves insulin sensitivity in pre-diabetic subjects.

Cinnamon, of course, has been a staple in many spicy dishes and enjoys its place as a health food. It is one of the most widely used spices in medicine and contains an array of phytochemicals that have been associated with both antioxidant properties and anti-inflammatory activity. The Chinese have often used Cinnamon as a treatment for type 2 diabetes. In this study, 30 non-diabetic patients were diagnosed with type 2 diabetes by a fasting blood glucose level of 126 mg/dl or higher (also known as impaired fasting glucose, or IFG). After six weeks of cinnamon supplementation, the patients reported an improvement in their blood sugar control. The patients who took two cinnamon capsules daily lowered their fasting blood glucose by an average of 10.37 mg/dl. Compared to the control group's results, this is a significant difference for the experimental group.

Gymnemic Acid

Gymnemic acid is an active component of the herb, Gymnema Sylvestre. It is a powerful inhibitor of intestinal glucose absorption in rats. It does so by stimulating the release of the hormone glucagon-like peptide-1 (GLP-1) from L cells in the intestine. Studies suggest that gymnemic acid could be a potential therapeutic option for diabetes treatment if GLP-1 levels can be increased naturally.

Genistein

Genistein, an isoflavone found in plants, possesses potent insulin-mimetic properties as well as anti-diabetic activity. It has been found to improve insulin sensitivity by activating the AMPK pathway and increasing glucose uptake into cells. An isoflavone extracted from soybeans, genistein, has also been found to have the ability to inhibit the peripheral process of hepatic gluconeogenesis. It was found that genistein significantly lowered blood glucose levels in diabetic mice by inhibiting hepatic gluconeogenesis. Another study published in the "Biochemical Pharmacology" journal discovered that genistein exhibits nootropic and neuroprotective properties against nerve cell death. It also prevents neuronal damage by increasing the activity of the brain-derived neurotrophic factor (BDNF) gene.

Berberine Hydrochloride

Berberine hydrochloride is a yellowish crystalline alkaloid obtained from various plants such as Coptis Chinensis, Hydrastis Canadensis, and Berberis vulgaris. It is an anionic isoquinoline alkaloid that has been used in traditional Chinese medicine for centuries. It is a known adaptogen that exhibits antioxidant, anti-inflammatory, immunomodulatory, and antiviral properties. It is a direct activator of AMPK (acetyl-CoA carboxylase) that triggers cellular lipid and glucose metabolism. It also has a major effect on cholesterol metabolism by increasing the production of HDL. It can improve insulin sensitivity through an increase in peripheral glucose uptake and release. This study conducted at Shandong University College of Traditional Chinese Medicine in China examined the effects of berberine hydrochloride on diabetic animal models and human subjects with T2D. The results showed that berberine had a positive effect on several processes associated with Diabetes, including impaired glucose tolerance, hyperglycaemia, hyperinsulinemia, and insulin resistance.

Polyphenols

Polyphenols are found in many plants, but especially those in the Mediterranean diet. Polyphenols are known for their antioxidant and anti-inflammatory activities. Green tea extract, for example, contains a high number of polyphenols, including epigallocatechin gallate (EGCG). A study published in the "Journal of Nutrition" found that EGCG was found to reduce oxidative stress-induced endothelial dysfunction by stabilizing nitric oxide activity. Another study published in the "Diabetologia" journal demonstrated that regular drinking of green tea significantly reduced insulin resistance and plasma glucose levels in a study of patients with type 2 diabetes. The tea polyphenols, specifically the catechins, were responsible for this effect.

Caffeine

It is hard to have a conversation about natural anti-diabetic remedies without mentioning the image of a steaming cup of coffee. Indeed, caffeine is one of the most commonly used natural remedies for high blood sugar levels. Caffeine has been known to improve glucose tolerance by increasing glucose oxidation in skeletal muscle and increasing fatty acid mobilization. It was found that caffeine ingestion increases glucose uptake by an insulin signal-independent pathway and improves insulin sensitivity in healthy non-obese men and women with impaired fasting glucose or impaired glucose tolerance. Coffee has also been shown to reduce glycated haemoglobin levels by -0.22% in patients with type 2 diabetes. The health benefits of coffee have been known for centuries, and it has been used as an alternative treatment for Diabetes for many years.

Resveratrol

Resveratrol is a stilbenoid and phytoalexin found in the skin of red grapes and other fruits such as mulberries, elderberries, and blueberries. It is well-thought-out as one of the most powerful polyphenols due to its antioxidant activity. It was discovered that resveratrol could inhibit glucose synthesis by stimulating peroxisome proliferator-activated receptors alpha (PPAR-alpha). This is a subtype of the nuclear hormone receptor that induces transcription via binding to specific DNA sequences. Resveratrol was also found to suppress tumour necrosis factor-alpha (TNF-alpha) activity, which has been implicated in developing insulin resistance.

Probiotics

The term "probiotic" refers to living microorganisms that provide health benefits to the host organism when ingested in adequate amounts. The most common probiotics include Lactobacillus and Bifidobacterium. Researchers have found that certain probiotics might benefit people with type 2 diabetes by improving insulin sensitivity.

CHAPTER 9:
THE BEST NATURAL INSULIN FOR TYPE 2 DIABETES

Type 2 diabetes is a chronic disease where the body can't produce or respond normally to insulin. Insulin is a hormone that regulates your blood sugar levels. When you have type 2 diabetes, you are constantly dipping into your energy reserves and lose fat from your muscles. This severely impedes future weight loss efforts and puts people with type 2 diabetes at risk for heart disease, kidney damage, nerve damage, stroke, depression and other problems. Obesity increases the risk of developing type 1 or type 2 diabetes, but it's not the only factor.

The following are some of the best natural insulin supplements:

Moringa Seed

(Store in the freezer)

Treatment of Diabetes is a very complex problem. It is very difficult to be sure that patients with type 2 diabetes are taking their medicine correctly. This is especially true of insulin. A great number of studies have revealed that many people with type 2 diabetes do not take their prescribed daily dose of insulin and often do not understand what they are supposed to be doing to take care of their condition. However, many people can produce insulin naturally and have been asked to use this way for general well-being. Moringa seed is one of the greatest natural insulin supplements.

Moringa is a tree common in Asia, Africa and Latin America. The leaves and pods are used as vegetables and can be ground into flour or used as tea. The seeds are edible too. Moringa has naturally occurring vitamins, minerals, and amino acids that can help prevent conditions like Diabetes, hypoglycaemia, obesity, etc. Moringa trees have been cultivated for centuries in many parts of the world where famine was common. Their leaves are full of natural nutrients that promote good health when consumed regularly.

Supplementing with moringa seeds has been shown to prevent the development of Diabetes in most people who took them regularly for at least a year.

Aframomum Melegueta

(Store in the refrigerator)

Aframomum melegueta is often called grains of paradise. It is a plant that grows in the tropical regions of Africa and thrives in sandy soils. The seeds are used medicinally and have been used for thousands of years for culinary and medical purposes. The seeds have been shown to lower blood sugar levels and improve insulin levels. They also reduce lipid peroxidation, inflammation and oxidative stress, which can prevent diabetes complications from occurring.

Berries

(Store in the freezer)

Berries are packed with antioxidants that can improve your health in many ways. In addition to antioxidants, berries are also full of fibre and other important nutrients. These nutrients can help decrease your overall risk of developing the disease, including Diabetes. Berries can also help you feel full and prevent overeating. This is important because when you have type 2 diabetes, your pancreas doesn't produce enough insulin. This causes blood sugar levels to increase, leading to hunger and cravings for sugary foods.

Phyllanthus Amarus

(Store in a cool, dry place)

Phyllanthus amarus has been used in traditional medicine in India for thousands of years to treat various health conditions like constipation, stomach problems and Diabetes. Research studies have revealed that it can recover insulin sensitivity and beneficial lipid profiles in the blood.

Myristica Fragans

(Store in the refrigerator)

The bark of this tree is what's used to make nutmeg. It has been used in traditional medicine for thousands of years to treat various health conditions like Diabetes, hypertension and respiratory issues like asthma. The bark contains antioxidants that can help prevent diabetes-related complications. In addition, a study conducted on rats showed that myristicin, a compound found in nutmeg, stimulated insulin secretion from pancreatic beta cells, which is crucial for the body's ability to regulate blood sugar levels.

Solanum xanthocarpum

(Store in a cool, dry place)

Solanum xanthocarpum is also known as the yellow mombin or gambooge. It is native to Central America and used the Maya to treat infection, diarrhea, fever and ulcers. According to research studies, it can help lower blood glucose levels. In addition, it has been shown to reduce cholesterol levels and body weight in rats.

Lagenaria Siceraria

(Store in the refrigerator)

Lagenaria siceraria is otherwise known as the bottle gourd or lauki. It is grown in India, Africa, Asia, Australia and North America. It is used for cooking purposes and as a diuretic. In Indian Ayurvedic medicine, it has been used to cure the following ailments:

It is recommended that one should chew the seeds of this gourd for better results.

Luffa Cylindrica

(Store in a dry place)

Luffa cylindrica or loofah is a herbaceous vine that belongs to the Cucurbitaceae family. It can be found in Africa, Asia and North America. It is widely used in beauty products because of its ability to remove dead skin cells and stimulate new cell growth. It is also used in Ayurvedic medicine to treat various conditions like arthritis, asthma, eczema, leukemia and Diabetes.

Momordica Charantia

(Store in the refrigerator)

Known as bitter melon is a vine a vegetable that's native to India. It has been shown to lower blood glucose levels in rats when taken regularly over an extended time. Bitter melon contains anthocyanins and other anti-diabetic compounds that have been shown to help prevent type 2 diabetes and reduce the risk of developing complications from insulin resistance.

Mangifera Indica

(Store in a cool, dry place)

Mangifera indica is native to tropical regions of Africa and Asia. It is cultivated commercially worldwide for its fruit which is eaten raw or used to make juice, candy and ice cream. In traditional medicine, it has been used to treat diabetes-like symptoms like inflammation and the sensation of thirst caused by high blood sugar levels.

Morus Alba

(Store in a cool, dry place)

Morus alba or mulberry contains antioxidants that have been shown to lower blood glucose levels in rats when taken regularly over an extended time. The leaves are likewise utilized in traditional medicine to treat blood disorders like anaemia and parasites.

Pinus koraiensis

(Store in the refrigerator)

Pine trees are native to China, Japan, Korea and Siberia and used for medicinal purposes for thousands of years. The bark of this tree has been used as a diuretic to treat diabetes-like symptoms of high blood sugar levels like thirst, frequent urination, fatigue and inflammation. In addition, the fruit is being studied for its ability to lower cholesterol levels and prevent heart disease.

Rosmarinus Officinalis

(Store in a cool, dry place)

Rosemary is a classic shrub that is natural to the Mediterranean. It is frequently used as a cooking herb and is widely consumed as a spice in cooking and Ayurvedic medicine. It has been used to treat digestive disorders, respiratory issues, depression, and even epilepsy in traditional medicine. It has also been revealed to advance insulin sensitivity to keep blood sugar levels under control.

Vitis Vinifera

(Store at room temperature)

Wine has been produced for the last 8,000 years, and wine grapes are one of the oldest domesticated plants on Earth. Wine is made from fermented grapes and has been used in traditional medicine to treat various health conditions. Studies have shown that wine can lower triglyceride levels in the blood and prevent heart disease. It also comprises antioxidants that can aid to lessen the risk of developing type 2 diabetes.

Withania Coagulans

(Store in a cool, dry place)

Withania coagulant is an Indian herb that has been used for thousands of years in Ayurvedic medicine to treat various health conditions, including Diabetes, cancer and respiratory issues like asthma. Research studies have also revealed its ability to improve insulin sensitivity to regulate blood sugar levels.

CHAPTER 10:
WHAT ARE THE BEST HEALTH SUPPLEMENTS FOR TYPE 2 DIABETES?

Maybe you've been using diabetes supplements for years and are looking for something new. Maybe your doctor has prescribed them, or maybe you want more information on the latest research. Whatever your case may be, we've got a comprehensive guide on the best supplements for type 2 diabetes and how they can help manage your blood sugar levels.

The following are some of the best health supplements for Type 2 Diabetes:

Vitamin D3

Vitamin D3 is essential for keeping your blood sugar levels stable. It also helps you absorb enough calcium, which gives you strength and holds your blood sugar balance.

How To Get Vitamin D3?

Vitamin D3 can be obtained from the Sun through exposure to sunlight or from your diet. When you are in the Sun, it triggers its conversion into Vitamin D3 by the skin. If you are doing a little bit of work outside, then get some natural sunlight, as this is necessary to produce Vitamin D3 in the body. If you live in areas where there is little sunlight or no natural sunlight, like U.S.A and Australia, then you can buy a Vitamin D3 supplement.

How to Take Vitamin D3 As a Type 2 Diabetic

The best way to take vitamin D3 is through an oral capsule. In this case, you would have to take a few supplements daily, and the capsule will keep them all in your bloodstream for many months. Some of these capsules are more expensive than others, but the price does not reflect quality, so we recommend buying from one of the best sellers.

Glucosamine

Glucosamine is a natural amino acid found in the body, and it's present in every part of our body, including the small intestines. It plays a vital role as it helps to maintain the proper functioning of nerves and cartilage in our joints.

As we age, our joints start to lose their natural lubricating properties. If we continue to age without glucosamine, we will eventually develop arthritis as well as other medical conditions, including Diabetes.

How To Take Glucosamine for Type 2 Diabetes

The best means is to purchase it online since it's easier to find a reputable vendor and a good selection. The dosage ranges depending on the brand you buy, but you will typically need to take anywhere from 500mg-1g of glucose-amine per day.

Cinnamon

A growing number of scientific studies conclude that Cinnamon can help manage blood sugar levels and boost metabolism. Some of the benefits are:

Reduces insulin resistance, which is why Type 2 Diabetics often need to increase or change their meds. Cinnamon has potency properties that help to regulate glucose production in the body. Medical studies have confirmed this effect, but on top of this, there are also numerous health benefits, such as lowering cholesterol and reducing inflammation in the body.

The best means to get the maximum of all the benefits is to go for a specific brand available online.

Chromium Picolinate

Of all the essential minerals required for the proper functioning of your body, chromium is one of the best. It's needed to activate certain enzymes required for sugar and fat metabolism, as well as protein synthesis and beneficial hormone production.

How To Take Chromium Picolinate for Type 2 Diabetes: The recommended dosage is 250-2000 mcg per day. The best means to learn what dosage works best is by visiting your local pharmacy or health store and asking a specialist for recommendations on which brand you should buy based on your needs and budget.

Vitamin D

This vitamin helps to regulate insulin levels in the blood. The best way to get this is through tanning, but many products contain Vitamin D that you can buy online or at your local pharmacy.

Zinc

Zinc is an essential mineral required for protein production and cell growth and repair in the body, and it's especially important for diabetics since it helps fight against oxidative stress that is present when Diabetes begins to progress.

Chlorella

Chlorella is a functional food that is high in protein and contains nine times the amount of chlorophyll than green vegetables and five times the amount of beta-carotene.

Amla

Amla is a potent antioxidant that helps to prevent cellular damage and slow down the aging process. It's rich in vitamin C, folic acid, vitamin E and other life-extending ingredients.

Berberine

Berberine extract is a natural plant compound that has numerous health benefits for many conditions, including Diabetes.

CHAPTER 11:
DIET FOR TYPE 2 DIABETES

Diabetes is a lasting sickness that distresses millions of Americans. It occurs when the pancreas produces too little insulin or when the body cannot use insulin as effectively as it should. The goal of diet management for type 2 diabetes aims to minimize blood sugar spikes and reduce the risk of diabetic complications.

Type 2 diabetes is connected with obesity, which leads to an increased risk of high cholesterol, high blood pressure, heart attack, stroke and kidney failure.

Foods To Eat for Person with Type 2 Diabetes

- Whole-grain breakfast cereals (shredded wheat, bran flakes, shredded wheat)

These can help to keep blood sugar stable and provide slow-release energy. Look for those high in fibre, like those containing whole wheat or rye

- Nuts

These are good snacks for people with Diabetes because they have a low glycaemic index. They also help lower cholesterol and provide omega-3 fatty acids, which are associated with a decreased risk of cardiovascular disease.

- Fish and lean meat

These should be served at least twice a week because they contain protein, which helps stabilize blood sugar levels. Choose lean cuts of meat, like chicken breast or turkey cutlets

- Fruits and vegetables

These should be eaten at least five times a day for maximum health benefits. They are rich in vitamins, minerals, fibre and antioxidants. They also help to improve blood sugar levels.
    o Blueberries, strawberries, raspberries

- Red/orange/yellow/green peppers
- Carrots
- Spinach
- Broccoli
- Kale
- Cauliflower

- Whole grains (brown rice, millet, etc.)

This can be included in the diet to maintain good health. However, they are not good for people with Diabetes because they tend to be high in starch and omitting them from the diet may lead to hypoglycaemia.

- Olive oil

Olive oil is filled with polyphenols in addition to monounsaturated fat. Studies have shown that olive oil may have anti-diabetic effects. Long-chain omega-3 fatty acids, originated in fish oils, also have been linked to improvement in glycaemic control and prevention of insulin resistance

- Legumes (beans, lentils)

They are high in protein and fibre. However, they are not recommended because their starch content can cause blood sugar spikes. They should be added to the diet only when pureed or ground into flour

- Fructose

This natural sweetener has been shown to lower blood sugar levels. However, it should be eaten in moderation because it may cause a rise in triglyceride levels

- Honey

Honey is a better choice for sweetening than sugar or artificial sweeteners because it consists of glucose and fructose. These are slowly absorbed into the bloodstream, which makes them good for people with Diabetes

- Dairy products (milk, yogurt)

These are recommended because they can keep blood sugar levels stable and contain calcium which can help to prevent osteoporosis. However, if you are lactose intolerant, it would be best to limit your consumption of dairy products

- Fish

Fish with great amounts of protein and omega-3 fatty acids may positively improve blood sugar control. However, some fish contain heavy metals such as mercury, which can cause problems

- Garlic

This spice has a magical reputation as a treatment for Diabetes. It is likewise rich in antioxidants that probably can reduce blood sugar levels. However, garlic preparations with high doses of sulphites should be avoided

- Anchovies

These small fish are rich in omega-3 fatty acids and antioxidants, which may benefit diabetic patients. However, they are high in sodium and low in calories, so they should be eaten strictly in moderation

- Tomatoes and tomatoes puree

These fruits may contain glucose that helps to stabilize blood sugar levels. The acids can also help reduce insulin resistance. However, the connection between tomatoes and blood sugar control has not been firmly established

- Parsley

This herb can lower blood sugar levels after meals and improve the elimination of uric acid, an element that stimulates the production of insulin

- Eggplant

Eggplants are rich in fibre, which helps to lower cholesterol levels and protect against heart disease. It also contains antioxidants, which may improve blood lipids

- Pumpkin

Pumpkin is a great source of beta-carotene and antioxidants, both of which play an important role in reducing the risk of Diabetes.

Foods To Avoid for People with Type 2 Diabetes

- Excessive consumption of refined grains (white bread; the more processed, the worse)

  These can lead to metabolic syndrome, which in turn can increase the risk of developing Diabetes.

- Excessive consumption of refined sugars (table sugar, high fructose corn syrup, etc.)

  This has been linked to the development of Diabetes and should be avoided. However, fruit juices may be just as bad as soft drinks because they are loaded with sugar and have no dietary fibre or protein.

- Refined vegetable oils (margarine; vegetable shortening)

  These promote the conversion of carbohydrates into fat. They also contain very little omega-3 fatty acids and can damage blood vessels. An even greater danger is the trans-fatty acids that they contain which cause heart disease and stroke

- Artificial sweeteners (sucralose, aspartame, etc.)
These can cause metabolic dysfunction and even Diabetes. The best choice is stevia.

- Alcohol
Extreme drinking of alcohol can increase the danger of Diabetes, so limiting it is recommended. However, there are healthier alternatives like red wine or green tea.

- Coffee
Coffee does not cause Diabetes, per se, but a study has found that long-term heavy consumption of coffee may increase the risk of developing the disease. However, this was based on small sample size. It is recommended to only drink coffee in moderation (1-2 cups/day).

- Nuts
These are high in omega-6 fatty acids and can damage blood vessels and cause metabolic syndrome if eaten in excess. However, moderate amounts of nuts do offer health benefits as they are rich in fibre, vitamins and minerals

- Excessive consumption of processed foods
These are low in nutritional value and often contain excessive amounts of salt and sugar. Such foods should be strictly avoided when trying to lose weight

- Excessive consumption of red meat
This can increase insulin resistance and lead to weight gain. It is recommended to cut back on red meat and eat more fish, nuts and legumes.

- Potatoes, yams and white rice
These are largely starchy and should only be eaten in small amounts with other foods that may be less harmful or even beneficial for Diabetes (fish, vegetables etc.)

- Food that is high in saturated fats
These have been linked to the development of Diabetes and are not recommended. However, some saturated fats like coconut oil and palm oil have been shown to lower cholesterol levels. It is also possible that they may lower the risk of diabetes, but more research is needed to confirm this.

- Fruit juices (they have a lot of sugar)

Juices contain a lot of sugar but no fibre or protein. The best choice would be pureed fruit or whole fruit + a small amount of juice (for example, apple + 5 ml juice per 5 apples). The fruit can be eaten separately if desired

- Soft drinks (they are linked to the development of Diabetes)

These are beverages with artificial sweeteners that have been linked to the development of Diabetes. It is best to avoid them altogether or replace them with unsweetened tea

- Vegetable oils (they have been shown to increase the risk of heart disease and stroke)

Vegetable oils contain trans-fatty acids that can damage blood vessels and increase the risk of stroke and heart attacks. It is best to avoid vegetable oils when possible.

- Processed meats (bacon, ham, sausages, etc.)

These can cause insulin resistance and increase the risk of Diabetes. However, unprocessed meats (beef, chicken) may be beneficial for diabetics and people at risk of developing Diabetes

- Sweetened condensed milk

This contains a lot of sugar and should be avoided. However, yogurt with low-carb sweeteners may not affect blood sugar levels

- Low-fat or fat-free foods

These are often high in carbohydrates and should be consumed in moderation. Dairy products like yogurt and cheese do have some health benefits for diabetics. However, low-fat dairy products may not be as healthy as their full-fat equivalents.

- Packaged snack foods

These are usually high in trans-fatty acids and should be avoided. The same goes for salty foods or any other type of junk food that is usually high in trans-fatty acids

- White potatoes or yams

These starchy foods are best consumed in moderation with other foods that may be less harmful or even beneficial for Diabetes (fish, vegetables etc.)

- High-glycemic foods (sweetened or unsweetened)

These are usually high in carbohydrates and should be avoided. However, some low sugar foods have been shown to decrease the risk of Diabetes. It is best to limit yourself to small amounts of these low-sugar foods per day and choose them carefully. See the food list below for recommendations.

- Sugar alcohols

These are often used as sweeteners in beverages such as diet sodas and sports drinks. The same goes for low-carb or natural carb sweeteners (erythritol, xylitol, lactitol etc.

- Pineapple

This is a good source of bromelain, which has been shown to help reduce blood glucose levels. The fruit also contains vitamin C and manganese, which is beneficial for diabetics. However, the leaves contain an insulin-like protein that may be harmful.

CHAPTER 12:
EXERCISE AND DIABETES

Type 2 diabetes is a long-lasting illness that needs to be managed daily. It's not always easy, but with a few careful choices, you can find ways to enjoy life without compromising your health. And when you exercise every day for 10 minutes, it becomes even more manageable.

Is It Safe for You to Exercise?

Significantly, you check with your doctor first. He or she can advise you about the proper diet and offer tips on how to improve your blood sugar levels.

The exercises in the following paragraphs will help you get started. But remember that maintaining good health involves a lot more than exercise alone. For example, if you smoke or have high cholesterol or high blood pressure, your doctor may recommend other treatments as well as exercise.

To keep a tight rein on your diabetes symptoms, it is important that you maintain a regular schedule of appointments with your doctor and keep careful track of all of your medications and symptoms.

The following are some of the exercises that can help you with your Diabetes:

Increasing Your Activity Level

The first goal is to increase your activity level. You can do this by:

- Going for a short walk during your break at work or during your lunch hour.
- Parking beyond away from the store or office.
- Walking the stairs instead of an elevator when you can.
- You are taking a walk after dinner and before bedtime. This will help you relax so that you sleep better and improve your blood sugar levels (this is helpful for people with type 1 diabetes as well).

- You were walking or jogging with a friend, neighbour, or co-worker who has Diabetes too. Work on improving each other's health. Share ideas about new ways to exercise and reach your goals more easily.

Taking It to the Next Level

The next step is to take it to the next level. How?

- Try swimming, biking, or working out in a gym.
- Adopt a new kind of exercises like weightlifting or aerobics classes. Try joining up for a class at your local gym or health club.
- Take your exercise outdoors—walking, jogging, or riding your bike for at least 20 minutes per day.

Covering Some Ground Daily

Deliberate daily movement is the key to healthy blood sugar control, according to the American Diabetes Association. Aim to cover at least 10,000 steps per day. For those who are very active, this might be as few as 2,000 steps.

Lifting Weights

Lifting weights is another great way to keep physically fit and boost your heart health. The goal with weightlifting is to use proper form so that the muscle groups you are working on do not fatigue too quickly and cause you pain or injury.

Exercise can help you lower your blood sugar levels by improving how your body processes sugar during exercise. During exercise, glucose is released into the bloodstream from the muscles and liver at a much faster rate than it would during rest or activity of any kind.

Weight Training

Weight training can help your muscles become more efficient at using glucose for energy. This is because the more often a muscle fibre is asked to contract, the stronger and more efficient it becomes. The best way to become stronger is by gradually increasing the weight you lift and the number of times you do this exercise during each session.

Perform Aerobic Exercise

Performing aerobic exercises such as running or walking helps improve endurance, lower blood pressure, raise HDL cholesterol levels, and help control weight gain. Aerobic exercise can also lower triglyceride levels in people with Diabetes, according to Johns Hopkins Medicine.

If you have been diagnosed with Diabetes, you should consult your physician about an exercise plan that will work for you. Your doctor may also recommend enrolling in a diabetes education class to learn more about the disease and effectively manage it with diet and exercise.

Yoga

Yoga is not just for people looking to become physically fit or improve their athletic performance, but it is also great for helping people control blood sugar levels. Yoga can aid you to relax and be more mindful of how your body feels when performing different activities, allowing you to better recognize when your blood sugar may be too low or too high.

Although many yoga classes involve a lot of physical activity, you don't have to be a gym rat to reap the benefits of this workout method. There are plenty of yoga videos and DVDs on the market that will help you learn how to do different poses at home, and it is important for patients with Diabetes to spend as much time in the Sun as possible. Sunlight is high in vitamin D, which helps regulate blood sugar levels and aid in weight loss. When practising yoga, it's also a great idea to wear sunscreen for added protection from harmful U.S. rays.

Pilates

Pilates is an exercise routine that uses small movements combined with deep breathing techniques to tone your entire body and increase flexibility. It helps diabetics control blood sugar levels and has been shown to increase the amount of insulin produced by the body.

Importance of Exercise to People with Diabetes

The study has revealed that regular physical activity helps people with Diabetes to maintain good blood sugar control. A study from the University of Buffalo found that people with type 2 diabetes performed better on a range of blood sugar tests after performing moderate exercise for a week than they did before starting the program.

Regular exercise helps to burn fat, which in turn lowers your blood pressure and cholesterol levels. A study from the Harvard School of Public Health found that men who engaged in regular aerobic exercise had a 4 per cent lower risk of suffering a heart attack or dying from heart disease than those who did not. Researchers noted that the type of exercise you do could make a difference as well. Although it was concluded that both endurance and resistance training were beneficial, it was found that the benefits were greater as the intensity (speed and weight) increased.

CONCLUSION

For all those who suffer from type 2 diabetes, you do have a natural cure. You can reduce or eliminate your chances of getting this disease by implementing these steps:

Let's start with lifestyle measurements.

- Stop eating fast foods and processed foods (stick to fresh food)
- Keep an eye on your blood sugar levels and make sure they are not too low or too high (close attention must be paid to this)
- Drink lots of water per day and keep hydrated. The good idea is to drink half your weight in ounces per day.
- Increase your fibre intake.
- Exercise at least 30 minutes per day, 5 days a week (more is better) Follow a strenuous activity that gets you breathing hard.
- Avoid alcohol and other drugs that increase blood sugar (like coffee and drugs to treat Diabetes).
- Avoid foods that increase your glucose levels (carbohydrates, sugar etc.).

So, let's try to make some changes in your life:

- Make sure you are eating no fast food or processed foods.
- Get lots of rest and sleep.
- Lift heavyweights at the gym to build muscles and stay healthy.
- Use a healthy diet, which is low in sugar and carbohydrates.
- Drink a lot of water during the day to keep your body hydrated and cleanse it from toxins and bad substances that are stored inside your body.
- Check glucose levels regularly, with a meter or by using strips, and make sure you don't eat too much sugar or carbohydrates since they will raise your blood sugar levels instantly if you have Diabetes or prediabetes (also avoid starch).

This book covers all the aspects of Diabetes in detail. It also explores the many different ways to control your blood sugar levels and the ways to prevent type 2 diabetes. In addition, it deliberates the cause of type 2 diabetes and its grave consequences. It also gives some methods for prevention, including diet and lifestyle factors that can help fight this disease.

Continually read this book if you want to avoid or cure type 2 diabetes!

The book describes how to use diet, exercise, medications and nutritional supplements to properly maintain your insulin levels. The book also provides a lot of valuable information regarding diabetes prevention.

It covers all the relevant information about Diabetes in a clear and precise manner. Here, you can also find information on diet and meal planning for Diabetes that will allow you to lose weight faster than ever before while nourishing your body with healthy food.

The book provides a lot of great tips on how to make your diet easier and more effective. The book also deliberates all the important issues related to diabetes medications and eating healthy on a budget. This book is full of valuable information for everyone who wants to become healthier and live longer!

Thank you for reading this book!

I hope this book was useful to you.

Good luck with your journey!

OTHER BOOKS WRITTEN BY RS JOHNSON

How to Overcome Depression: How to Remove Depression, Anxiety, and Addiction
https://www.amazon.com/dp/B0971QXBXH
Digital Product creation
https://www.amazon.com/dp/B098J4VPJF
How to Launch a Digital Product Business
https://www.amazon.com/dp/B098KFTF1S
NLP For Beginners
https://www.amazon.com/dp/B098JBH28Q
Credit Repair Secrets
https://www.amazon.com/dp/B098KMQY36
All You Need to Know About Cryptocurrency Understanding Risk And Reward In Investing
https://www.amazon.com/dp/B099P1XCWQ
Eliminating Your Debt in 12 (x) Easy Steps and Keep Them Off: A Practical Guide To Eliminating Your Debt Forever!

https://www.amazon.com/dp/B099P4BT47
Taking full charge of your finance: Easy Guide to Personal Finance
https://www.amazon.com/dp/B099P6B7HH
Sure Steps to Wealth Creation: How to Build Wealth From Nothing
https://www.amazon.com/dp/B099P53K5T
How to Find the Best Home Business that fits Your Needs: Starting A Business QuickStart Guide
https://www.amazon.com/dp/B09CD775HQ
How to Cure Erectile Dysfunction without Drugs: The Absolute Guide on How to Cure ED
https://www.amazon.com/dp/B09CGBCTY7
How to Develop Excellent Communication Skills: Communication Skills Training
https://www.amazon.com/dp/B09CD8H55N
Be A Fat-Burning Machine: The Metabolism Advantage
https://www.amazon.com/dp/B09CD8WXT2
All You Need To Know About Car Insurance: The Inside Secrets Of Car Insurance
https://www.amazon.com/dp/B09CD8SGSR
How To Save Money On Airfare: How To Travel For Cheap
https://www.amazon.com/dp/B09CDFDZZ4
Simple Ways To Have A Balanced Mental Health: How To Improve Mental Health

21 Days Practical weight Loss Program
Achieve result in 14 days with Green Tea diet
Acne Removal, achieve a smooth babylike skin
Appling Keto diet effectively for maximum result
Body detox that works****
Destroy blood pressure naturally before it destroys you.
Diabetic diet that brings result
Food that heals
Getting result from Vegan diet, the proper way
Getting result with TLC diet
Gluten free diet the right way
Keto Diet
Keto diet and intermittent fasting
Losing weight without fasting
Low carb diet, get result in 21 days
Natural cure for type 2 diabetes
One meal a day with paleo diet, surest way to lose weight
Proper way to buttock diet
Raw food diet with it benefits
Thyroid diet cookbook
Diet that keeps your blood pressure down
Effective pregnancy diet
Food that slows aging process and their applications
Juicing for health